Big Guy Weight Loss

Exactly How to Lose 40, 80 or Even 100+ Pounds

By Daniel Falcon

Disclaimer and Terms of Use:

We have made effort to ensure that the information in this book is accurate and complete. However, the author do not warrant the accuracy of the information, text and graphics contained within the book due to the dynamic nature of science, research, known and unknown facts and internet. The Author does not hold any responsibility for omissions, errors, or misinterpretation of the information in the book. This book is presented solely for motivational and informational purposes only. Consult your doctor before trying anything in this book.

Table of Contents

Introduction

Being overweight is a world epidemic with very serious consequences. It does not discriminate gender or age and affects all in equal measure. Those who are very heavy usually suffer in silence and are usually discriminated against, especially when it comes to job opportunities; they are usually left out, either because of their physical looks or because there are certain types of jobs that they can't do, especially those that require high mobility. People who are overweight are also psychologically traumatized because they are often faced with rejection in whichever groups they try to fit in. Those who are overweight are usually referred to as being obese. Obesity is a heavy accumulation of fat in the body to an extent that it increases an individual's risk of diseases that can damage their health and reduce their lifespan.

To know whether you are obese, you need to work out your Body Mass Index (BMI). You can calculate your BMI by dividing your weight by the product of your height by itself, i.e. BMI = $\frac{Weight}{Height \ x \ Height}$ kg/m^2. The table below can help you know whether you have a normal weight or you are obese.

	Normal	Overweight	Obese	Very Obese
BMI	19 – 24	26 – 29	30 – 39	40 and above

Apart from the physical and psychological challenges, obesity also has medical challenges that can even lead to death! Some of these challenges include diabetes, heart diseases and many more.

The medical treatments of these diseases are very expensive and may even include bariatric surgery. In extreme cases, the treatments may even fail to work! That's why you wouldn't want to fall a victim of any of these conditions.

If you are very heavy (extremely obese) and are struggling with your weight, there are weight loss intervention programs that combine exercise and diet can really work for you. The benefits of exercise have been known for so many years, but research now shows that lifestyle changes can have positive impact on people who are very heavy.

This is great news to these people since it means that those who cannot afford medical treatments now have this cheaper option. And that is what this book is all about.

Mindset for Successful Weight Loss

To help understand the mindset for successful weight loss we must first of all mention something about the mindset that leads to weight gain. And after discussing the mindset for successful weight loss, we will put to you the mindset you should have once you have achieved your weight loss goal so you don't slip again.

But what exactly do we mean by mindset? Mindset can be defined as a set of fixed ideas or attitudes that someone has and that are usually difficult to change. It can also be used to describe a combination of an individual's worldview about a subject, any beliefs and biases, and particularly the habits that attach to those beliefs.

In this section we are going to explore the changing mindsets of those who are successful in lasting weight loss:

a) as they were putting on weight
b) as they were trying to change and trying to lose weight so as to achieve their target weight
c) as they adapted to their new weight and started witnessing their mindset change

The question we need to ask ourselves when it comes to food is whether it is belief or habit that comes first. Perhaps you have never thought about it, but just ate something repeatedly until you got into the habit, and so you subconsciously thought that it was alright. It is also like when you planned to drive somewhere after work, but just found yourself driving home automatically, meaning you had got into the habit of driving home. This analogy is exactly what happens when it comes to food choices. You will realize that it is the habit that rules and no conscious decision is made.

The mindset that leads to weight gain

The mindset tat leads to weight gain is a melting pot of two ingredients: false beliefs and mindlessness. False beliefs about food and drinks are usually based upon thinking that certain foods are good for you but in the actual sense, they help your body to store fat. Mindlessness is when you just eat whatever food you want or whatever food is available, not being consciously aware of your food choices. In simple terms, this mindset means you don't give a thought about what goes into your mouth.

The mindset during the start of the weight loss process

This mindset comes in when you have realized that you are overweight and have decided to do something about it. It is the time you will become willing to be taught and to trust the teacher plus the weight loss program suggested. If you have accepted the program, your teacher can tailor it to suit your condition to give you confidence to employ a positive mindset.

There are usually certain fears that you will need to overcome as you jump into the weight loss program taken. Some people fear failing, while surprisingly enough, some fear succeeding. But the good news is that all humans have fears whenever it comes to issues dealing with any change process. So just take the fears as normal and take one step at a time. Just set your mind that you can achieve your goal just like other people have done so.

The mindset once a person's weight loss goal has been achieved

While still undergoing the weight loss process, you will be having some conscious decisions and actions about food and exercise choices. But once you achieve your goal, these conscious actions and decisions will be transformed into habits and rituals. They will now be coming out naturally without much struggle. But still, there will be some forces within your mind and body that will try to drag you back. Some environmental forces involving places and people may also try to drag you back, so you will need to stay conscious of your new habits and rituals.

When the weight loss program you chose has given you a positive result, it is advisable to stick to it no matter what other people say. The truth of the matter is that those who have been successful have discovered what is good for their body and mind. And what is right for one person may not be right for another, so keep in mind that the well-meaning pieces of advice that someone might give you are based on what they perceive to be right for them.

As you embark on the journey to weight loss, be aware of your current mindset and the change process, and be willing to ask for help along the way.

Workout Routines

Your body needs physical exercise to stay healthy. Exercise offers benefits that even dieting can not offer. It turns your body into a fat blasting furnace and boosts your metabolism. There is no weight loss program that can be without a workout routine because it speeds up the whole weight loss process. There are different workout plans that you can choose from. Here we are going to discuss a day-to-day workout plan and a 6-week workout routine. All these routines should involve both cardiovascular exercise and resistance training.

Day-by-day workout routine

This routine takes between 4 and 12 weeks depending on how much weight you want to lose. Combine this workout routine with portion control and healthy eating to enable you to lose weight effectively. If you do so, you will be able to burn at least a pound or two of body fat per week.

Cardiovascular exercise

This exercise is centered around the cardio and is able to burn a lot of calories.

Steady-state cardio (or simply "cardio") is an exercise which involves working out at about the same level of intensity for the duration of the exercise. The exercise may involve running, power walking, cycling, jogging, etc. It tends to take a long time.

Cardiovascular interval training (IT) is a shorter workout that alternates between higher levels of intensity and recovery intervals. It is the perfect technique to torch body fat and massively boost metabolism.

Cardiovascular high intensity interval training (HIIT) is more or less like IT but involves more intense form of interval training like sprinting.

As a beginner you can start with regular interval training but make sure that it is something you enjoy doing so that you don't give up along the way. If you have cardiovascular machinery, you can do the workouts indoors otherwise do them outdoors. And if you are carrying a lot of weight, it is advisable to start with low impact exercises such as swimming, walking or using the elliptical machine. The elliptical machine is great as it allows you to burn as many calories as you would do while running or jogging, and using it is easier.

Cardiovascular exercises get progressively harder as you move from one level of workout plan to the next. This is to make you stronger and fit and also to ensure that you keep losing weight. As you do a particular exercise over and over again, it will eventually become easier, this means your body will no longer require working hard and you will be burning less calories. That's why every week you should try to do better than the previous week.

Resistance training

Resistance training focuses on building the muscle. During an exercise, not all weight that is lost is fat, some of it is muscle. So this training will ensure that you don't lose muscle but instead build them. You will be required to do 3 resistance workouts per week, including abs and back (core), upper body and total body workout. You can follow these exercises by a short cardio workout to maximize fat burning.

For this training, you will only need some basic equipment like a resistant band, a stability ball and two pairs of dumbbells – a light pair (5 – 10lb) and a heavy pair (10 – 20lb).

Beginner to Advanced Workouts

Workout plans are there for beginners and for more advanced exercisers. In case you have not exercised for a long time, start with the beginner workout plan. You can then proceed to the intermediate workout plan and finally to the advanced workout plan.

Before you start a new exercise program, check with your doctor especially if you have a medical condition and remember to warm up for 5 to 10 minutes before you start the workout and also to stretch after the workout.

The following are the suggested workout plans for various levels.

12 WEEKS							
	MON	TUE	WED	THU	FRI	SAT	SUN
WEEK 1	Core workout	20-30 min cardio	Upper body workout	20 – 30 min cardio	Total body workout	20 – 30 min cardio	Rest
WEEK 2	Core workout	30 min cardio	Upper body workout	30 min cardio	Total body workout	30 min cardio	Rest
WEEK 3	20 min cardio	30 – 40 min cardio	Upper body workout	30 – 40 min cardio	Total body workout	30 – 40 min cardio	Rest
WEEK 4	Core workout then 20 min cardio	40 – 45 min cardio	Upper body workout	40 – 45 min cardio	Total body workout	40 – 45 min cardio	Rest
WEEK 5	Core workout then 20 min cardio	45 min cardio	Upper body workout	45 min cardio	Total body workout	20 min IT	Rest
WEEK 6	Core workout then 20 min cardio	45 min cardio	Upper body workout	45 min cardio	Total body workout	20 min IT	Rest

15

12 WEEKS (…continued)

	MON	TUE	WED	THU	FRI	SAT	SUN
WEEK 7	Core workout then 10 min IT and 10 min cardio	45 min cardio	Upper body workout	45 min cardio	Total body workout	20 min IT	Rest
WEEK 8	Core workout then 15 min IT and 10 min cardio	45 min cardio	Upper body workout	45 min cardio	Total body workout	20 min IT	Rest
WEEK 9	Core workout then 15 min IT and 10 min cardio	45 min cardio	Upper body workout then 15 min IT and 10 min cardio	45 min cardio	Total body workout	45 min cardio	Rest
WEEK 10	Core workout then 15 min IT and 10 min cardio	45 min cardio	Upper body workout then 15 min IT and 10 min cardio	45 min cardio	Total body workout	45 min cardio	Rest
WEEK 11	Core workout then 15 min IT and 10 min cardio	45 – 60 min cardio	Upper body workout then 15 min IT and 10 min cardio	45 – 60 min cardio	Total body workout	45 – 60 min cardio	Rest
WEEK 12	Core workout then 20 min IT and 10 min cardio	45 – 60 min cardio	Upper body workout then 20 min IT and 10 min cardio	45 – 60 min cardio	Total body workout	45 – 60 min cardio	Rest

16

Intermediate Workout Plan

				12 WEEKS				
	MON	**TUE**	**WED**	**THU**	**FRI**	**SAT**	**SUN**
WEEK 1	Core workout	30 – 40 min cardio	Upper body workout	30 – 40 min cardio	Total body workout	30 – 40 min cardio	Rest
WEEK 2	Core workout	45 – 60 min cardio	Upper body workout	45 – 60 min cardio	Total body workout	45 – 60 min cardio	Rest
WEEK 3	Core workout then 20 min cardio	45 – 60 min cardio	Upper body workout	45 – 60 min cardio	Total body workout	45 – 60 min cardio	Rest
WEEK 4	Core workout then 20 min cardio	50 – 60 min cardio	Upper body workout	50 – 60 min cardio	Total body workout	50 – 60 min cardio	Rest
WEEK 5	Core workout then 20 min cardio	45 – 60 min cardio	Upper body workout then 20 min cardio	45 – 60 min cardio	Total body workout	45 – 60 min cardio	Rest
WEEK 6	Core workout then 15 min HIIT and 10 min cardio	45 min cardio	Upper body workout then min HIIT and 10 min cardio	45 min cardio	Total body workout	45 min cardio	Rest

12 WEEKS (...continued)

	MON	TUE	WED	THU	FRI	SAT	SUN
WEEK 7	Core workout then 15 min HIIT and 10 min cardio	45 min cardio	Upper body workout then min HIIT and 10 min cardio	45 min cardio	Total body workout	45 min cardio	Rest
WEEK 8	Core workout then 20 min HIIT and 10 min cardio	45 min cardio	Upper body workout then 20 min HIIT and 10 min cardio	45 min cardio	Total body workout	45 min cardio	Rest
WEEK 9	Core workout then 20 min HIIT and 10 min cardio	45 – 60 min cardio	Upper body workout then 20 min HIIT and 10 min cardio	45 – 60 min cardio	Total body workout	45 – 60 min cardio	Rest
WEEK 10	Core workout then 20 min HIIT and 10 min cardio	45 – 60 min cardio	Upper body workout then 20 min HIIT and 10 min cardio	45 – 60 min cardio	Total body workout	45 – 60 min cardio	Rest
WEEK 11	Core workout then 20 min HIIT and 10 min cardio	45 – 60 min cardio	Upper body workout then 20 min HIIT and 10 min cardio	45 – 60 min cardio	Total body workout then 20 min cardio	45 – 60 min cardio	Rest
WEEK 12	Core workout then 20 min HIIT and 10 min cardio	45 – 60 min cardio	Upper body workout then 20 min HIIT and 10 min cardio	45 – 60 min cardio	Total body workout then 20 min cardio	45 – 60 min cardio	Rest

Advanced Workout Plan

		MON	TUE	WED	THU	FRI	SAT	SUN
	12 WEEKS							
		MON	TUE	WED	THU	FRI	SAT	SUN
WEEK 1		Core workout	45 – 60 min cardio	Upper body workout	45 – 60 min cardio	Total body workout	45 – 60 min cardio	Rest
WEEK 2		Core workout	60 min cardio	Upper body workout	60 min cardio	Total body workout	60 min cardio	Rest
WEEK 3		Core workout then 20 min cardio	60 min cardio	Upper body workout then 20 min cardio	60 min cardio	Total body workout	60 min cardio	Rest
WEEK 4		Core workout then 20 min cardio	60 min cardio	Upper body workout then 20 min cardio	60 min cardio	Total body workout	60 min cardio	Rest
WEEK 5		Core workout then 20 min HIIT	60 min cardio	Upper body workout then 10 min HIIT and 10 min cardio	60 min cardio	Total body workout	60 min cardio	Rest
WEEK 6		Core workout then 15 min HIIT and 10 min cardio	60 min cardio	Upper body workout then 15 min HIIT and 10 min cardio	60 min cardio	Total body workout	60 min cardio	Rest

12 WEEKS (...continued)

	MON	TUE	WED	THU	FRI	SAT	SUN
WEEK 7	Core workout then 20 min HIIT and 10 min cardio	60 min cardio	Upper body workout then 20 min HIIT and 10 min cardio	60 min cardio	Total body workout	60 min cardio	Rest
WEEK 8	Core workout then 20 min HIIT and 10 min cardio	60 min cardio	Upper body workout then 20 min HIIT and 10 min cardio	60 min cardio	Total body workout	60 min cardio	Rest
WEEK 9	Core workout then 20 min HIIT and 10 min cardio	60 min cardio	Upper body workout then 20 min HIIT and 10 min cardio	60 min cardio	Total body workout then 20 min cardio	60 min cardio	Rest
WEEK 10	Core workout then 20 min HIIT and 10 min cardio	60 min cardio	Upper body workout then 20 min HIIT and 10 min cardio	60 min cardio	Total body workout then 10 min HIIT and 10 min cardio	60 min cardio	Rest
WEEK 11	Core workout then 20 min HIIT and 10 min cardio	60 min cardio	Upper body workout then 20 min HIIT and 10 min cardio	60 min cardio	Total body workout then 10 min HIIT and 10 min cardio	60 min cardio	Rest
WEEK 12	Core workout then 20 min HIIT and 10 min cardio	60 min cardio	Upper body workout then 20 min HIIT and 10 min cardio	60 min cardio	Total body workout then 10 min HIIT and 10 min cardio	60 min cardio	Rest

This routine stimulates as much fat loss as possible; it consists of 3 full body workouts per week, 2 days of cardiovascular workouts and 2 days of rest.

6 WEEKS							
	MON	**TUE**	**WED**	**THU**	**FRI**	**SAT**	**SUN**
WEEK 1	Full body workout	Cardio workout	Full body workout	Rest	Full body workout	Cardio workout	Rest
WEEK 2	Full body workout	Cardio workout	Full body workout	Rest	Full body workout	Cardio workout	Rest
WEEK 3	Full body workout	Cardio workout	Full body workout	Rest	Full body workout	Cardio workout	Rest
WEEK 4	Full body workout	Cardio workout	Full body workout	Rest	Full body workout	Cardio workout	Rest
WEEK 5	Full body workout	Cardio workout	Full body workout	Rest	Full body workout	Cardio workout	Rest
WEEK 6	Full body workout	Cardio workout	Full body workout	Rest	Full body workout	Cardio workout	Rest

Nutrition fundamentals

There are plenty of ways to lose weight; the problem only arises when you have to maintain your weight loss over a long period of time. Maintaining that weight you have worked hard to achieve requires that you be careful with what you eat. Maintaining a healthy weight for the rest of your life is all about energy balance. Here are 3 basic steps you can follow to succeed.

Make smart choices from every food group

Your body needs the right fuel for your stress-filled, hectic schedule. You therefore need to enjoy a wide variety of nutrient-rich foods packed with protein, energy, vitamins and minerals. It is suggested that you go for whole grains from bakery, fruits and vegetables, lean proteins and low-fat products.

Get the most nutrition from your calories

Eating smarter does not mean that you have to go fat-free and sugar-free immediately. You can just eat and drink smaller portions and make empty calories choices less often that will make a big difference in your calorie intake.

The key here is to moderate not to eliminate. For example, you can drink water instead of sugary drinks, eat desserts less often and watch your portion sizes.

Balance Food and Physical Activity

For you to lose weight you need spend more calories in your daily activities than you take. Fit more activity into your daily life to help burn more calories. Follow the workout routines suggested in the previous section.

Being Too Strict

Dieters usually make a mistake of going into a diet with the intention of being overly strict on what they eat. But the problem comes when they slip up; they see it as absolute failure and quit the entire program, going back to the bad, old habits. You need to approach dieting with a flexible mindset. Allow yourself to have food, here and there, that is inconsistent with your program once in awhile. Otherwise, you may drive yourself nuts and may be end up worse that when you started.

Are Carbs Really the Enemy?

Carbs are not that bad, unless you eat large amounts of high glycemic index (GI) carbs. This is because they result in higher amounts of blood glucose which leads to higher levels of insulin after their ingestion. High levels of insulin have been related to increased fatness because insulin is the body's main anabolic hormone, increasing fat stores, protein stores and glycogen stores.

Sources of high GI carbs include refined sugar and refined starch e.g. cereals, potatoes, white bread, popcorn, rice, carrots, etc. Sources of low GI carbs include fruits and all vegetables excluding carrots. Although carrots are high on the GI, you would have to consume a large amount of it daily in order to get the full effect as you would from a normal serving of high GI carbs.

Fibers

Fibers can be water insoluble or water soluble. Soluble fibers are rapidly broken down and fermented unlike the insoluble fibers. For that reason they slow the appearance of glucose in the blood due to their viscous property. They therefore aid in lowering the blood concentrations of ingested macronutrients resulting to lower amounts of absorbed energy. Sources of soluble fiber include wheat, psyllium, melons, whole-grain breads, oat bran, etc.

Eat Fat

That sounds interesting, but it's the truth. Fats are a vital part of a diet. There are two types of fats: saturated fats and unsaturated fats. Diets that are high in saturated fats should be avoided because they keep lipolytic enzymes dormant hence promote fat stores. Sources of saturated fats include cookies, margarines, most snack foods, crackers etc. Unsaturated fats (oils) are a healthy source of fat when taken in moderate or low amounts. Without them, your body will not function properly. Sources of unsaturated fats (oils) include flaxseed oil, soybean oil, olive oil, salmon, safflower oil, peanuts, wall nuts, cod, sunflower oil, tuna, etc.

Protein

This is the only macronutrient with a Recommended Daily Allowance (RDA), and it is 0.8 grams per kilogram of body weight. Athletes may benefit from increasing protein intake to between 1.2 and 1.6

grams of protein per kilogram of body weight. But it should be noted that excess protein is stored as fat meaning they can also make you fat. If you increase your protein intake, you should also increase your water intake so as to keep your kidneys healthy. The best sources of protein are usually in the form of animal tissues such as chicken, beef, fish, soy bean, etc.

RECIPES

These simple calorie-burning recipes will help you lose weight very fast. The recipes include at least one weight-loss superfood and they can be made in 30 minutes or even less! We make it easy with our satisfying, healthy options for breakfast, lunch and dinner.

Breakfast Recipes

Chocolate and Peanut Butter Smoothie

Ingredients

3/4 cup frozen berries

1/4 cup low-fat vanilla yogurt

1/2 cup low-fat chocolate soy milk

2 tablespoons reduced-fat all-natural peanut butter

Directions:

Place all of the ingredients into a blender and blend until smooth and creamy. Stop and stir when necessary. Serve immediately.

Ingredients

3 egg whites

Whole-grain English muffin

1/2 cup spinach

1 slice reduced-fat cheddar cheese

1 slice tomato

Directions

Step 1: Scramble 3 egg whites.

Step 2: Cover half of a whole-grain English muffin with 1/2 cup spinach and the other half with 1 slice reduced-fat cheddar cheese

Step 3: Toast until cheese is melted

Step 4: Add egg and 1 slice tomato.

Ingredients

1 packet plain, instant oatmeal

1/2 cup skim milk

3/4 of a small apple, chopped

1 teaspoon cinnamon

1 teaspoon brown sugar

1 tablespoon chopped walnuts

Directions

Step 1: Prepare 1 packet plain, instant oatmeal with 1/2 cup skim milk

Step 2: Microwave 3/4 of a small apple, chopped, 1 teaspoon cinnamon, and 1 teaspoon brown sugar

Step 3: Top oatmeal with apples and 1 tablespoon chopped walnuts

Ingredients

3 egg whites

1/4 cup canned black beans

1 ounce reduced-fat cheddar cheese

 2 tablespoons salsa

Directions:

Step 1: Scramble 3 egg whites with 1/4 cup canned black beans (rinsed and drained) and 1 ounce reduced-fat cheddar cheese

Step 2: Top with 2 tablespoons salsa

Ingredients

Whole-grain bagel

1 tablespoon reduced-fat all-natural peanut butter

1 apple, sliced

Directions:

Step 1: Toast the whole-grain bagel

Step 2: Spread with 1 tablespoon reduced-fat all-natural peanut butter

Step 3: Cover with apple slices

Turkey-Avocado Melt

Ingredients

2 to 3 slices roasted turkey

2 slices avocado

1 slice low-fat pepper jack cheese

2 slices whole-grain bread

Directions:

Step 1: Place 2 to 3 slices roasted turkey, 2 slices avocado, and 1 slice low-fat pepper jack cheese between 2 slices whole-grain bread

Step 2: Grill in skillet

Ingredients

1/2 cup whole wheat pasta

1 cup sauteed spinach

2 tablespoons pine nuts

2 tablespoons low-fat feta

Capers and chopped sun-dried tomatoes

Directions:

Step 1: Toss 1/2 cup cooked whole wheat pasta with 1 cup sauteed spinach and 2 tablespoons each pine nuts and low-fat feta

Step 2: Sprinkle with capers and chopped sun-dried tomatoes

Guacamole Burger

Ingredients

Veggie burger

An avocado

1/2 cup salsa

A whole-grain bun

Directions

Step 1: Cook a veggie burger according to package directions

Step 2: Mash half an avocado with 1/2 cup salsa

Step 3: Top burger with avocado mixture

Serve on a whole-grain bun

Ingredients

1/2 cup udon

1 cup spinach

1 1/2 cups hot vegetable broth

1/2 cup cubed tofu

1/2 cup chopped mushrooms

1 teaspoon soy sauce

Directions:

Step 1: Combine 1/2 cup cooked udon with 1 cup spinach and 1 1/2 cups hot vegetable broth

Step 2: Add the 1/2 cup cubed tofu, 1/2 cup chopped mushrooms, and finally the 1 teaspoon soy sauce

Ingredients

1/3 cup tomato sauce

1 naan

 2 cups spinach

1/4 cup low-fat mozzarella cheese

1 tablespoon slivered almonds

Directions:

Step 1: Spread 1/3 cup tomato sauce on 1 naan

Step 2: Top with 2 cups spinach, 1/4 cup low-fat mozzarella cheese, and 1 tablespoon slivered almonds

Step 3: Bake at 350 degrees F until melted

Ingredients

1/2 cup black beans

1/2 chopped bell pepper

Chopped onion

1 chopped jalapeno

2 teaspoons olive oil

Brown rice

1/4 avocado

Directions:

Step 1: Cook 1/2 cup each black beans, chopped bell pepper, and chopped onion and 1 chopped jalapeno in a pan with 2 teaspoons olive oil for 5 minutes

Step 2: Place over cooked brown rice

Step 3: Top with 1/4 sliced avocado

Ingredients

3 ounces chopped chicken

2 tablespoons crumbled low-fat blue cheese

1/2 cup chopped cucumber

1 tablespoon chopped pecans

1 tablespoon dried cranberries

2 cups lettuce

2 tablespoons vinaigrette

Directions:

Step 1: Place 2 tablespoons crumbled low-fat blue cheese, 3 ounces chopped chicken, 1/2 cup chopped cucumber, and 1 tablespoon chopped pecans and chopped and dried cranberries on 2 cups lettuce

Step 2: Toss with 2 tablespoons vinaigrette

Chicken Salad with Citrus Dressing (Warm)

Ingredients

4 medium sized chicken breast halves (without bones or skin) – about 1 pound
1 1/2 ounce chicken broth
2 1/2 cups strawberries
1/3 cup orange juice
2 tablespoons salad oil
2 tablespoons lemon peel, shredded
1 teaspoon sugar
1/2 teaspoon chili powder
1/4 teaspoon salt
1/4 teaspoon freshly ground black pepper
6 cups torn spinach or other greens
Makes: 4 servings

Directions:

Step 1: Sprinkle the chicken-breast halves lightly with salt and pepper.

Step 2: Pour chicken broth into a large saucepan; add chicken. Bring broth to a boil; reduce heat. Cover and simmer for 15 to 20 minutes, or until chicken is tender and no longer pink. Remove chicken from broth with a slotted spoon and cool slightly.

Step 3: Combine the half cup of the strawberries, orange juice, salad oil, lemon juice, sugar, lemon peel, chili powder, black pepper and salt. Blend until smooth then transfer to a small saucepan and boil. Uncover then simmer for 5 minutes while stirring occasionally.

Step 4: Thinly slice chicken breasts. In a large bowl, toss together salad greens, remaining strawberries, and chicken.

Step 5: To serve, drizzle warm dressing over salad. Sprinkle with walnuts.

Ingredients
1/2 medium avocado, seeded and peeled
1 tablespoon lime juice
Salt
Ground black pepper
2 slices whole wheat bread, torn
3 tablespoons fresh cilantro leaves
2 garlic cloves
1 15-ounce can black beans, rinsed and drained
1 canned chipotle pepper in adobo sauce
2 teaspoons adobo sauce
1 teaspoon ground cumin
1 beaten egg
1 small plum tomato, chopped

Makes: 4 servings

Directions:
Step 1: In a small bowl, mash the avocado. Stir in lime juice then season to taste with salt and pepper. Cover this and chill until ready to serve.
Step 2: Place torn bread in a food processor. Cover and process until bread turns into coarse crumbs. Transfer to a large bowl; set aside.
Step 3: Place the garlic and cilantro in the food processor. Process after covering until finely chopped then add the chipotle pepper, beans, cumin and adobo sauce.

Step 4: You can then add this mixture to bread crumbs followed by the egg.

Step 5: Lightly grease the rack of a grill pan. Place patties on the rack. Cook over medium-high heat for 8 to 10 minutes, or until patties are heated through, turning once.
Step 6: To serve, top patties with guacamole and tomato.

Ingredients

12 ounces chicken breast strips (without bones or skin)

1/4 teaspoon garlic salt

1/8 teaspoon black pepper

Nonstick cooking spray

2 cups packaged broccoli slaw

1/2 teaspoon ground ginger

3 tablespoons creamy peanut butter

1 tablespoon reduced-sodium soy sauce

1/2 teaspoon minced garlic

3 10-inch whole wheat tortillas, warmed

Makes: 6 servings

Directions:

Step 1: Sprinkle chicken strips with garlic salt and pepper. Coat a skillet with cooking spray. Add chicken; cook over medium-high heat for 2 to 3 minutes, or until no longer pink. Remove from pan; keep warm. Add broccoli and 1/4 teaspoon of the ground ginger to skillet. Cook and stir for 2 to 3 minutes, or until vegetables are crisp-tender.

Step 2: In a saucepan, combine peanut butter, 2 tablespoons water, soy sauce, minced garlic, and the remaining ginger then heat over low heat while whisking constantly until smooth,.

Step 3: To assemble, spread tortillas with peanut sauce. Top with chicken strips and vegetable mixture. Roll up each tortilla, securing with a toothpick. Cut in half; serve immediately.

Ingredients

1/2 cup uncooked quinoa

1 cup water

2 Roma tomatoes, seeded and finely chopped

1/2 cup shredded fresh spinach

1/3 cup finely chopped red onion

2 tablespoons lemon juice

2 tablespoons olive oil

1/2 teaspoon salt

Spinach leaves

2 avocados, peeled, pitted and sliced

1/3 cup crumbled feta cheese

Makes: 4 servings

Directions:

Step 1: Boil water and quinoa in a small saucepan. Cover and simmer for 15 minutes after reducing thee heat.

Step 2: Stir quinoa, tomatoes, spinach, and onion together in a bowl.

Step 3: Whisk together oil, lemon juice, and salt then mix with quinoa.

Step 4: Place avocado slices and spinach on plates with and quinoa then sprinkle with feta.

Closing Remarks

We hope you have enjoyed reading the book and are now ready to make an informed decision. The book has covered everything you need to know about losing weight if you are extremely obese. It has discussed what obesity is, how you can determine whether you are obese or not, and the risks you face if you are obese. The section on workout routines is very comprehensive and has presented a 12-week workout plan for beginners, a 12-week intermediate workout plan, a 12-week advanced workout plan and a 6-week fat-burning workout plan.

Another interesting part of the book is the nutrition fundamentals where you are advised on how you can get the best out of each food group. This section has also discussed how best you can balance between exercise and food. Finally, the book gives you some recipes that are great for weight loss.

We now believe that you appreciate the fact that losing weight is about having the right mindset, and combining both exercise and healthy eating.

We wish you well on your journey to a normal weight.

www.ingramcontent.com/pod-product-compliance
Lightning Source LLC
Chambersburg PA
CBHW072019290526
45787CB00013B/1354